# *Healing Plates: A Guide to Anti-Inflammatory Meal Prep*

*A non stress meal plan with easy recipes to heal the immune system, prep and recipes for long term healing.*

*Dr Robert Anderson*

# Copyright

# Introduction

- *Healing Plates: A Guide to Anti-Inflammatory Meal Prep"* is a culinary compass navigating the intersection of wellness and gastronomy. Authored with precision and passion, this book transforms mealtime into a therapeutic experience. Immerse yourself in a journey that goes beyond the kitchen, delving into the profound impact of anti-inflammatory nutrition on overall health. The pages unfold a tapestry of delicious recipes, seamlessly blending flavour and healing properties. From vibrant salads to hearty entrees, each dish is a celebration of ingredients specifically curated to combat inflammation. This guide not only empowers readers with practical meal prep techniques but also enlightens them on the profound influence of food choices in fostering well-being. Prepare to embark on a transformative gastronomic expedition that revitalises the body and delights the palate.

# Table Of Contents

# Introduction And Brief overview of inflammation and its impact on health.

Inflammation is the body's natural response to injury or infection. It involves immune cells, blood vessels, and molecular mediators. While acute inflammation is crucial for healing, chronic inflammation can negatively impact health. It's linked to various conditions, including cardiovascular diseases, autoimmune disorders, and neurodegenerative diseases. Lifestyle factors like diet, stress, and lack of exercise can influence inflammation levels. Maintaining a balanced lifestyle and addressing underlying health issues are key to managing inflammation for overall well-being.

# Chapter 1

***The Prelude to Inflammation.*** "The Prelude to Inflammation" could delve into the initial events and signals that set the stage for inflammation to occur in the body. It might explore factors such as tissue damage, microbial invasion, or the release of signalling molecules like cytokines and chemokines. The chapter could also discuss how the immune system detects these triggers and initiates the inflammatory response, highlighting the roles of various cells and molecules involved in the process. Additionally, it might touch upon the distinction between acute and chronic inflammation and the implications for health and disease. Overall, Chapter 1 could lay the foundation for understanding the intricate mechanisms that underlie inflammation and its importance in the body's defence and pathology.

# Chapter 2

# The Ant-inflammatory Diet

In the quest for well-being, a path unfolds, paved with choices that echo through the corridors of our bodies. Welcome to the realm of the anti-inflammatory diet—a symphony of foods orchestrated to cultivate balance and quell the fires of inflammation.As we journey through this chapter, envision a plate adorned with the vibrant hues of nature's bounty. Fruits, vegetables, and whole grains take centre stage, each morsel a tribute to the intricate dance between nutrition and inflammation.Picture the graceful arcs of omega-3-rich fish navigating through the sea of choices. These fatty acids, like skilled navigators, chart a course toward a state of equilibrium within our bodies. Meanwhile, healthy fats play their part, offering a nourishing embrace that whispers tales of cellular harmony.Yet, in this gastronomic voyage, there are adversaries to be mindful of—processed foods, sugar, and the siren call of saturated fats. They lurk in the shadows, ready to disrupt the delicate equilibrium we seek.This culinary odyssey is not merely a trend but a mindful embrace of the profound connection between what we consume and how our bodies respond. As we delve into the chapters that follow, let this be a foundation—an invitation to explore the art of nourishing oneself with intent and reverence.But, dear reader, remember always to seek the counsel of those versed in the language of health. The journey toward well-being is unique for each, and guidance from healthcare professionals ensures a path aligned with individual needs.As we turn the page, let us embark on this gastronomic expedition, savouring the flavours of a life in tune with the anti-inflammatory symphony—a melody composed by the choices we make, echoing through the corridors of our own well-being.

# Chapter 3

## Principles of anti-inflammatory diet

In the tapestry of health, Chapter 3 unfolds the principles of the anti-inflammatory diet, a symphony of choices that orchestrates well-being. Picture a canvas adorned with vibrant fruits, crisp vegetables, and the subtle hues of omega-3-rich fatty fish. This chapter delves into the essence of an anti-inflammatory lifestyle, where every bite is a brushstroke contributing to the masterpiece of vitality.As our journey begins, we encounter the protagonists—fruits and vegetables, bursting with micronutrients and antioxidants. They stand as guardians against the forces of inflammation, offering a bounty of vitamins and minerals that fortify the body's defences. Through their vivid colours and natural goodness, they weave a narrative of resilience and nourishment.In the anti-inflammatory saga, nuts and seeds play a crucial role, providing a wholesome dose of essential fatty acids. Like ancient treasures, they bestow the gift of omega-3s, crucial allies in the battle against chronic inflammation. These healthy fats, akin to magical elixirs, dance through the bloodstream, soothing the fires of inflammation and promoting balance.Our narrative takes a turn towards the briny depths as we encounter fatty fish—salmon, mackerel, and sardines. Rich in omega-3 fatty acids, these aquatic marvels swim against the current of inflammation, embodying the principle of choosing foods that heal from within. Their presence in the anti-inflammatory diet is akin to a maritime alliance, safeguarding against the tempest of chronic inflammation.Yet, no tale is complete without acknowledging the shadows on the culinary stage. Refined sugars and saturated fats emerge as the antagonists, casting a veil of inflammation upon our protagonists. This chapter urges a conscious departure from processed temptations, guiding readers away from the treacherous path that leads to the heart of inflammation.In the intricate narrative of Chapter 3, the anti-inflammatory diet emerges as a holistic approach, a lifestyle choice that transcends mere sustenance. It beckons us to partake in a culinary journey where every morsel contributes to the symphony of health—a melody of balance, vitality, and resilience against the discordant notes of inflammation.

## Chapter 4

# Emphasising whole, nutrient-dense foods

Emily's kitchen became a haven of health as she delved into the art of anti-inflammatory meal preparation. Every ingredient was a brushstroke on the canvas of her well-being, and each meal was a step toward healing from within.In the quiet moments of chopping vibrant vegetables and sizzling sound of sautéing, Emily discovered the therapeutic power of crafting her own nourishment. Gone were the days of mindless eating; in its place emerged a deliberate, intentional approach to food.The chapter of anti-inflammatory meal prep began with an exploration of the colourful spectrum of fruits and vegetables. Emily reveled in the antioxidants of blueberries, the anti-inflammatory properties of leafy greens, and the earthy goodness of turmeric. Her pantry transformed into a treasure trove of healthful delights, stocked with quinoa, wild-caught salmon, and olive oil—the foundation of her anti-inflammatory plate.Meal prep, once a chore, evolved into a meditative practice. Emily marinated proteins with anti-inflammatory herbs and spices, visualising the healing journey each bite would embark upon within her body. As the aroma of roasted vegetables wafted through her kitchen, Emily felt a profound connection to the earth's bounty and the nurturing power it held.With each carefully planned meal, Emily discovered the joy of variety and the pleasure of savouring wholesome flavours. Breakfasts adorned with fresh berries and chia seeds, lunches featuring colourful salads with a sprinkle of nuts, and dinners showcasing grilled vegetables and lean proteins—all orchestrated to create a symphony of wellness on her plate.The healing journey extended beyond the kitchen. Emily's newfound energy and vitality became her companions, guiding her through the demands of daily life. Friends noticed the glow in her complexion, and Emily shared the secret of her transformative chapter—the healing plate.In this culinary voyage, Emily not only nourished her body but also cultivated a profound understanding of the intimate connection between food and well-being. As Chapter 4 unfolded, Emily realised that the healing plate was not just a collection of ingredients; it was a testament to her commitment to a life of balance, health, and vibrancy.

# Chapter 5

## Anti-inflammatory Ingredients

In the pursuit of well-being, unlocking the secrets of anti-inflammatory ingredients has become a journey into the heart of nature's healing arsenal. This chapter delves into the potent elements that have emerged as key players in the quest for a balanced and inflammation-free life.Turmeric: The Golden HealerWithin the vibrant hues of turmeric lies curcumin, a compound celebrated for its anti-inflammatory prowess. Joining hands with centuries-old traditions, this golden spice has woven itself into the fabric of holistic healing, offering a natural remedy to soothe the body and mind.Ginger: Nature's ElixirAs another gem in nature's treasure trove, ginger reveals its anti-inflammatory magic. From ancient apothecaries to modern kitchens, this versatile root has been a steadfast ally, known for alleviating inflammation and promoting digestive harmony.Omega-3 Fatty Acids: Nourishing from the DepthsEmbarking on a journey to the depths of the sea, omega-3 fatty acids emerge as guardians of wellness. Found in the depths of fish oil and flaxseeds, these fatty acids stand as pillars of anti-inflammatory support, encouraging a resilient and responsive body.Green Tea: Elixir of SerenitySteeped in tranquillity, green tea unveils its anti-inflammatory essence. Rich in antioxidants and catechins, this ancient brew extends its soothing touch, encouraging a state of calmness while combating inflammation.Vitamin D: The Sunshine NutrientBathed in sunlight, vitamin D takes centre stage as a vital component in the anti-inflammatory narrative. From bone health to immune resilience, this sunshine nutrient orchestrates a symphony of well-being, ensuring inflammation finds no foothold.Quercetin: Antioxidant HarmonyIn the colourful realm of fruits and vegetables, quercetin stands out as an antioxidant virtuoso. With a brushstroke of anti-inflammatory finesse, this plant compound paints a picture of cellular harmony, fortifying the body against inflammatory storms.As we explore these chapters in nature's healing manuscript, it becomes evident that the key to well-being often lies in the simplicity of what the Earth generously offers. In embracing these anti-inflammatory allies, we embark on a journey towards a harmonious coexistence with our bodies and the natural world.

# Chapter 6

## Breakfast Bliss

As the sun rises, casting its gentle glow across the morning sky, there's no better way to greet the day than with a nourishing breakfast. In this chapter, we'll explore a variety of healing recipes designed to kickstart your day with delicious flavours and wholesome ingredients.1. Energising Acai BowlIngredients:1 frozen banana.

1/2 cup frozen mixed berries.

1/4 cup unsweetened almond milk.

1. packet frozen acai pureeToppings of choice: sliced fruit, granola, shredded coconut, chia seeds. Instructions:In a blender, combine the frozen banana, mixed berries, almond milk, and acai puree. Blend until smooth and creamy.Pour the mixture into a bowl and top with your favorite toppings such as sliced fruit, granola, shredded coconut, and chia seeds.

2.Protein-Packed Quinoa Breakfast BowlIngredients:

1/2 cup cooked quinoa.

1/4 cup Greek yogurt,                1 tablespoon honey,              1/4 teaspoon cinnamonToppings of choice: sliced banana, chopped nuts, drizzle of almond butter.

Instructions:

In a bowl, combine the cooked quinoa, Greek yoghourt, honey, and cinnamon. Mix well to combine.Top the quinoa mixture with sliced banana, chopped nuts, and a drizzle of almond butter.
3.Veggie-Packed Breakfast Burrito Ingredients:
2 large eggs, beaten.              1/4 cup diced bell peppers.       1/4 cup diced tomatoes.          1/4 cup chopped spinach 2 whole wheat tortillas
Optional toppings: avocado, salsa, shredded cheese

Instructions:

In a skillet, scramble the eggs over medium heat until cooked through.Add the diced bell peppers, tomatoes, and chopped spinach to the skillet. Cook for an additional 2-3 minutes until vegetables are tender.Divide the egg and vegetable mixture between the two whole wheat tortillas. Add optional toppings such as avocado, salsa, and shredded cheese if desired. Roll up the tortillas into burritos and serve.These breakfast recipes are not only delicious but also packed with nutrients to fuel your body and mind for the day ahead. Whether you prefer a refreshing acai bowl, a protein-packed quinoa breakfast bowl, or a savoury breakfast burrito, there's something here to satisfy every craving and kickstart your morning on the right foot.

*Chapter 7: **Customising Your Meal Plan.*** In this chapter, we delve into the art of tailoring your meal plan to suit your unique needs, preferences, and health goals. From adapting recipes for dietary restrictions to making sustainable changes for long-term health, here's everything you need to know to create a meal plan that works for you.Tailoring Your Meal PlanNo two individuals are the same, so why should their meal plans be? It's essential to customise your meal plan to fit your lifestyle, dietary requirements, and personal preferences. Whether you're aiming to lose weight, gain muscle, or simply maintain a healthy lifestyle, a personalised meal plan is key to success.Adapting Recipes for Dietary Restrictions or Food AllergiesLiving with dietary restrictions or food allergies doesn't mean you have to compromise on flavour or nutrition. With a bit of creativity and the right substitutions, you can still enjoy delicious meals that cater to your needs. Learn how to adapt recipes to accommodate gluten intolerance, lactose intolerance, nut allergies, and other dietary restrictions without sacrificing taste or variety.Making Sustainable Changes for Long-Term Health. A successful meal plan isn't just about short-term results—it's about making sustainable changes that promote long-term health and well-being. Discover how to incorporate nutritious whole foods, balance macronutrients, and practice mindful eating habits for lasting success. By focusing on gradual, sustainable changes, you'll not only achieve your health goals but also maintain them for years to come.Whether you're a seasoned meal planner or just starting out on your journey to better health, customizing your meal plan is essential for success. With the tips and strategies outlined in this chapter, you'll be well-equipped to create a meal plan that nourishes your body, satisfies your taste buds, and supports your long-term health goals.

# Chapter 8: Lifestyle Factors for Managing

InflammationInflammation is a natural response of the body to injury or infection, but when it becomes chronic, it can lead to various health issues. Fortunately, there are lifestyle factors that can help manage inflammation effectively. In this chapter, we will explore three crucial aspects: stress management and relaxation techniques, incorporating physical activity into your daily routine, and getting quality sleep for optimal health and inflammation management.1. Stress Management and Relaxation Techniques:Chronic stress can trigger inflammation in the body, so it's essential to find ways to manage stress effectively. Incorporating relaxation techniques such as deep breathing exercises, meditation, yoga, or mindfulness can help reduce stress levels and lower inflammation. Taking breaks throughout the day to engage in activities you enjoy, spending time in nature, or practising gratitude can also contribute to overall stress reduction.2. Incorporating Physical Activity into Your Daily Routine:Regular physical activity is not only beneficial for cardiovascular health and weight management but also plays a significant role in reducing inflammation. Aim for at least 30 minutes of moderate exercise most days of the week. This could include activities such as walking, cycling, swimming, or strength training.

Find activities that you enjoy and make them a part of your daily routine to reap the anti-inflammatory benefits.3. Getting Quality Sleep for Optimal Health and Inflammation Management:Quality sleep is essential for overall health and well-being, including inflammation management. Aim for 7-9 hours of uninterrupted sleep each night. Establishing a regular sleep schedule, creating a relaxing bedtime routine, and optimizing your sleep environment can help improve sleep quality. Avoiding caffeine, electronic devices, and stimulating activities before bedtime can also promote better sleep.In conclusion, lifestyle factors such as stress management, regular physical activity, and quality sleep play crucial roles in managing inflammation effectively. By incorporating these practices into your daily routine, you can support your body's natural ability to reduce inflammation and promote overall health and well-being.

# Chapter 9: Embracing a Healthier, Anti-Inflammatory

LifestyleCongratulations on reaching the end of your anti-inflammatory meal prep journey! Throughout this book, you've learned valuable strategies and techniques for incorporating anti-inflammatory foods into your diet to promote overall health and well-being. As you reflect on your progress and achievements, take a moment to celebrate the positive changes you've experienced.Reflecting on Your Progress and AchievementsThink back to when you first started your anti-inflammatory journey. Perhaps you were experiencing chronic pain, digestive issues, or fatigue. Now, take stock of how far you've come. Have you noticed improvements in your symptoms? Are you feeling more energised and vibrant? By committing to an anti-inflammatory lifestyle, you've taken a proactive step towards better health, and that's something to be proud of.Celebrating Positive ChangesCelebrate the victories, no matter how small they may seem. Whether it's fitting into an old pair of jeans, enjoying a restful night's sleep, or simply feeling more mentally alert, each positive change is a testament to your dedication and perseverance. Take time to acknowledge and celebrate these achievements—they are milestones on your journey to vibrant health.Looking Ahead to a Future Filled with Vibrant Health and VitalityAs you continue on your anti-inflammatory journey, keep your eyes focused on the future. Visualize yourself living a life filled with vibrant health, vitality, and joy. Imagine waking up each day feeling refreshed and rejuvenated, ready to tackle whatever challenges come your way. By staying committed to your anti-inflammatory lifestyle, you're laying the foundation for a healthier, happier future.Appendix: Additional ResourcesTo support you on your journey, we've compiled a list of additional resources for further exploration of anti-inflammatory nutrition. Whether you're looking for more recipe inspiration, meal planning tools, or wellness support, these resources are here to help you along the way.Recommended reading: Explore these books for in-depth information on anti-inflammatory nutrition and its benefits.Websites and apps: Discover online resources and mobile apps that offer meal planning assistance, recipe inspiration, and support from the anti-inflammatory community.Glossary of terms: Refer to this glossary for definitions of key terms related to inflammation and nutrition, helping you better understand the science behind your dietary choices.As you close this chapter and continue on your journey towards better health, remember that you have the power to shape your own destiny. Embrace the principles of anti-inflammatory nutrition, stay motivated, and

never lose sight of your goals. Your body will thank
you for it.

*Healing Plates: A Guide to Anti-Inflammatory Meal Prep" offers* a comprehensive approach to improving health through mindful eating. By emphasising anti-inflammatory ingredients and meal prepping strategies, the book empowers readers to take control of their well-being. Through its insightful guidance and delicious recipes, it encourages a lifestyle centred around nourishing the body and promoting healing from within. As the journey to optimal health continues, "Healing Plates" serves as a valuable resource and a beacon of hope for those seeking balance and vitality in their lives.